For permission requests, contact Keisha McDonald-Griffin at AmourLegacipublishing@gmail.com

This is a work of non-fiction. Any resemblance to actual events or persons, living or dead, is entirely coincidental. This manual is designed to provide factual information and instructions that may present real world details and procedures.

1st editionBook Design: Keisha McDonald-Griffin
Production: AmourLegaci Publishing
Editing: Keisha McDonald
Illustration: Keisha McDonald-Griffin
Publisher: AmourLegaci Publishing
To order: Amazon.com
Author Website:Amourlegacipublishing.com
Printed in United States of America

Flow and Glow

Note from the Therapist!

Hey there! Growing up comes with lots of changes, and you are doing an amazing job. Remember, you are strong, beautiful, and so capable! You've got this, and you are never alone. Shine bright and be kind to yourself!

♥ – Keisha McDonald, LPC

Chapter 1: Understanding Your Period

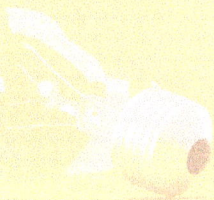

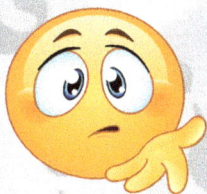

What's the Deal with Periods?

Alright, let's talk periods—not the ones at the end of a sentence, but the kind that show up once a month and make you wonder, Wait, what is happening to my body?!

First things first: getting your period is completely normal! It means your body is growing up and working the way it's supposed to. It might seem weird or even a little scary at first, but once you understand what's going on, you'll feel way more confident and in control.

Here's the big picture:

Every month, your body prepares for the possibility of a baby **(don't worry, this doesn't mean you're having one anytime soon!).**
It does this by creating a soft, cushiony lining inside your uterus—kind of like making a cozy bed. But if no baby is needed, your body says, Welp, don't need this right now! and releases that lining.

That's what your period is—it's just your body letting go of that extra lining, which comes out as a mix of blood and tissue through your vagina. This happens about once a month, and it's totally normal!

The Menstrual Cycle
(AKA Your Body's Monthly Routine)

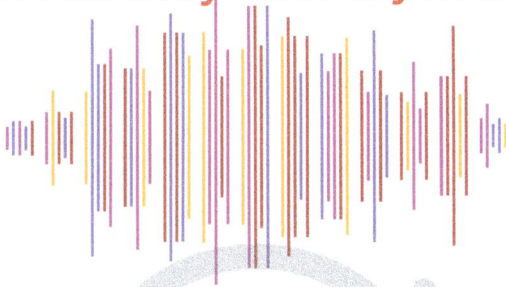

Your period is just one part of a cool, monthly cycle that your body follows. Think of it like a playlist on repeat, but instead of songs, it's different phases your body goes through every month!

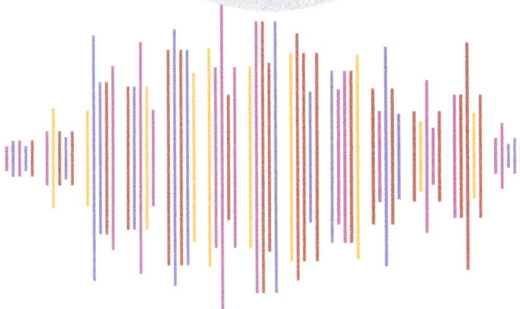

Here's the breakdown:

🎵 Track 1:
The Beginning Phase
(Days 1-7)

This is when your period happens.
Your body is clearing out the old lining, and you might see red, brown, or pinkblood when you go to the bathroom. It usually lasts 3 to 7 days.

🎵 Track 2:
The Prep Phase
(Days 8-14)

After your period ends,
your body starts building a fresh new lining inside your
uterus—just in case it's needed.

Here's the breakdown continued:

🎵 Track 3:
The Ovulation Phase
(Around Day 14-16)

Your ovary releases an egg
(you won't feel this happening!).
This is just part of your body's natural cycle.

🎵 Track 4:
The Waiting Phase
(Days 17-28)

If the egg isn't needed,
your body gets ready to clear out the lining
again—which means your period is on its way,
and the cycle starts over!

Most menstrual cycles last about 28 days, but some are
shorter (21 days) or longer (up to 35 days). That's totally
okay! Every girl's cycle is a little different, and that's normal.

What You Might Feel
(AKA Period Symptoms!)

Your body is working hard during your period, and sometimes that means you'll feel some changes in your body and mood.

Here's what to expect:

Physical Symptoms
(Your Body's Way of Saying "Hey, I'm Working Here!")

✅ **Cramps** — That achy, twisty feeling in your lower belly? That's your uterus doing little squeezes to push out the old lining. A heating pad, stretching, or deep breathing can help!

✅ **Bloating** — Your stomach might feel a little puffy or tight (like when you eat a big meal). Drinking water helps!

✅ **Breast Soreness** — Your chest might feel a little tender or sensitive. Totally normal, and it goes away!

✅ **Headaches** — Some girls get mild headaches before or during their period. Staying hydrated and getting rest helps.

Emotional Symptoms
(Because Hormones Have a Mind of Their Own!)

Mood Swings — One minute you're laughing, the next you're annoyed at your pencil for existing. It's the hormones talking!

Feeling Extra Emotional — You might feel like crying over a cute puppy video (or a commercial about cereal—no judgment!).

Low Energy — Your body is busy doing important work, so you might feel more tired than usual. Take it easy and get good sleep! Not everyone feels all these symptoms, and they can be different each month. The good news? You can manage them!Things like staying hydrated, eating healthy snacks, moving your body, and getting enough rest can help you feel way better.

Hormones

Meet Your Inner Messengers—The Hormones!
Welcome to the Secret HQ of YOU!

Hey there, superstar! 🌟
Did you know your body has tiny, invisible messengers running around, sending secret signals to help you grow, feel, and even start your period? Yep! These little messengers are called hormones—and they are like a squad of superheroes working behind the scenes.

Hormone HQ: Where the Magic Happens
Imagine your brain has a control center—kind of like the headquarters in a spy movie! 🕵️
Inside, a tiny but mighty boss called the pituitary gland is making big decisions. It tells your body, "Alright, time to start changing!" and BOOM—hormones rush out like excited messengers, delivering their notes to different parts of your body.

Meet the Squad:
The Key Players in Puberty!

🚀 Estrogen – The super-planner!
It helps your body grow, shapes your curves, and gets your uterus ready for periods. Think of it as the architect of your body's big changes.

🔥 Progesterone – The cozy creator!
It works with estrogen to help with your period cycle and make sure your body stays balanced. It's like a gentle coach, making sure everything runs smoothly.

⚡ Testosterone – The energy booster!
Even though it's more famous for boys, girls have a little bit too! It helps with muscle growth, energy, and even mood. Think of it as a secret power-up!

The Secret HQ of YOU!

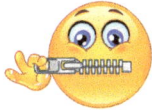

Why Do Hormones Make You Feel... ALL THE FEELS?

One minute you're laughing, the next you feel like you might cry over a cute puppy video. 😭🐶

What's up with that?

Well, hormones also send signals to your emotions. It's like having a radio station in your brain that sometimes plays happy tunes and other times plays dramatic movie soundtracks.

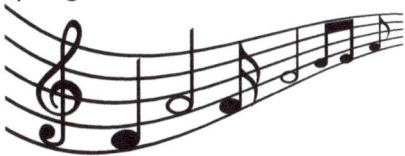

The Secret HQ of YOU!

How to Work WITH Your Hormones
(Not Against Them!)

🛏️ **Get Sleep:** Your body needs rest to keep everything balanced.
(Yes, beauty sleep is real!)

🥦 **Eat the Rainbow:** Fruits, veggies, and proteins give your hormones the fuel they need.

💃 **Move Your Body:** Dancing, stretching, or just wiggling around helps shake off stress.

The Secret HQ of YOU!

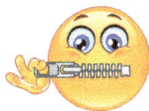

Why Do Hormones Make You Feel... ALL THE FEELS?

One minute, you're laughing at a meme. The next, you're tearing up over a cute puppy video. And then—BOOM—you're suddenly annoyed because your favorite snack is GONE! 😭🍪

What's up with that?!

Well, your hormones are like tiny DJs in your brain, switching up the music on your feelings playlist without warning! Sometimes they play a fun, upbeat song, and other times, it's a slow, emotional ballad. 🎵🎶

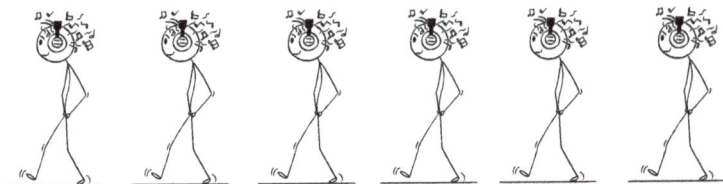

The Secret HQ of YOU!

How to Work WITH Your Hormones
(Not Against Them!)

Here's how hormones can shake things up:

💓 **Mood Swings:** Estrogen and progesterone can make your emotions more intense—like turning up the volume on everything you feel. One day, you might feel super confident, and the next, you're questioning everything.
(Totally normal, BTW!)

🍕 **Cravings & Energy Ups & Downs:** Ever suddenly want ALL THE CHOCOLATE 🍫 or feel super tired for no reason? Hormones can affect hunger and energy levels, making you crave certain foods or feel extra sleepy.

The Secret HQ of YOU!

How to Work WITH Your Hormones
(Not Against Them!)

😡 **Irritation Station:** Sometimes, things that normally don't bother you suddenly do **(like your sibling breathing too loud! 🤯).**

This is because your brain is adjusting to new hormone levels, and it takes time to get used to them.

😊 **Super Happy, Super Sad, Super Everything:**
Puberty is like riding a roller coaster with surprise loops! 🎢
You're not just happy—you're SO HAPPY! And when you're sad, it can feel like
THE SADDEST SAD EVER.
The good news?
These feelings pass, and you learn to ride the wave. 🌊

QUIZ TIME!!!

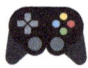

🎮 Fun Game:

The Hormone Roller Coaster! 🎢
Let's see how well you can match
hormones to emotions and
actions!

👉 **How to Play:**

Below are different situations. Pick the hormone that might be at work!

1 You suddenly feel like hugging your best friend for no reason.

A) Estrogen

B) Testosterone

C) Progesterone

2 You're STARVING and could eat a whole pizza by yourself. 🍕

A) Progesterone

B) Estrogen

C) Sleepy-time Hormones

3 You feel super confident and ready to take on the world. 💪

A) Estrogen

B) Testosterone

C) Progesterone

4 You cry during a commercial about baby animals. 🐶

A) Estrogen

B) Happy Hormones

C) Stress Hormones

5 You feel super sleepy and just want to curl up in a blanket. 😴

A) Estrogen

B) Progesterone

C) Jumping Beans Hormone

The Most Important Thing to Remember

Your period is not a **big scary monster**—it's just a normal, natural part of life. It means your body is growing and doing exactly what it's supposed to do.

And guess what? You're not alone. Millions of girls and women experience this every day. The more you learn about your cycle, the more confident you'll feel.

So, deep breath—you got this! 💖

(Answers: 1-A, 2-A, 3-B, 4-A, 5-B)

Next up:

NEXT »

How to take care of yourself during your period!

Chapter 2: What to Expect

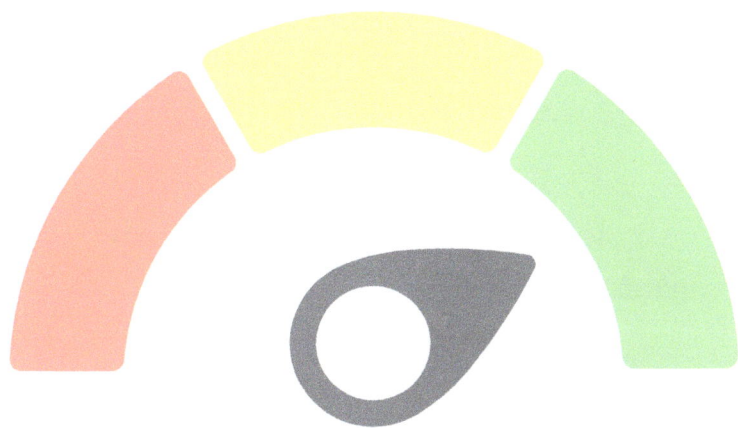

EXPECTATIONS

How to Recognize When Your First Period is Coming

Alright, so you're wondering when your first period will arrive.
Is there a giant calendar in the sky that tells you?
Not exactly, but your body does give you hints that your period might be on its way!

Here are some clues to look for:

Discharge – A clear or white fluid in your underwear? That's called discharge, and it usually starts six months to a year before your first period.

Mood Swings – One minute, you're excited, and the next, you feel annoyed for no reason. Hormones are at work!

Body Changes – You might notice hair growing under your arms and in your private areas.

Breast Changes – Your chest might feel a little sore or start growing.

Every girl is different, so don't stress if your friends start before you or after you. Your body is on its own schedule!

How Long Does a Period Last & What's Normal?

Your first few periods might be a little unpredictable. One month it might last 3 days, another month 7 days—and that's totally normal!
Most periods last between 3-7 days, and in the beginning, they might not come every month.

Your body is figuring things out, just like you are!

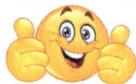

Period Tracking Basics

Think of period tracking like keeping score in a game—except this game helps you understand your body better!

You can track:

- **When your period starts and ends**
  (so you can predict when it'll come next)
- **How heavy or light it is**
  (use a scale from ☁ to ⛈)
- **Symptoms**
  (like cramps, bloating, or mood swings)

You can use a journal, an app, or even a simple calendar.

Tracking helps you stay prepared and know what's normal for **YOU**!

Chapter 3: Managing Your Period

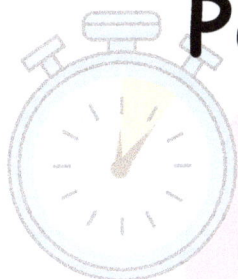

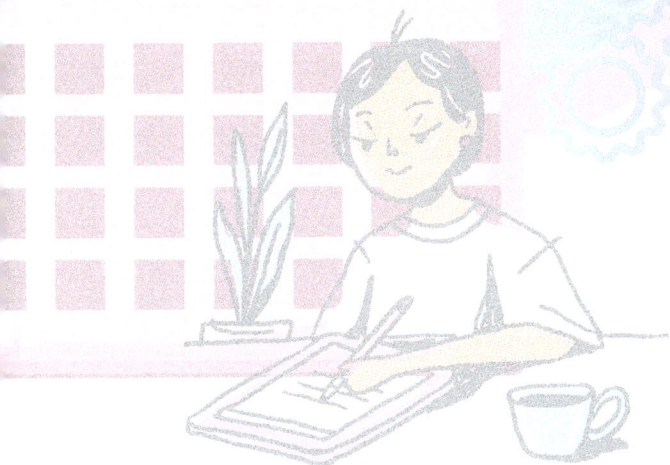

How to Use
Pads, Tampons & Period Underwear

You've got options!

Here's a quick breakdown:

- **Pads** 🩸 — Stick them inside your underwear. Change every 4-6 hours **(or sooner if it's full!)**

- **Tampons** 🩹 — Inserted into the vagina, they soak up blood from the inside. Change every 4-8 hours. Start with small sizes until you're comfortable.

- **Period Underwear** 🩲 — Looks like regular underwear but has built-in protection. Great for light days or backup!

Try different products to see what works best for you—there's no wrong choice!

Dealing with Leaks & Accidents

Oops! Had a little leak? No big deal! It happens to everyone.

Here's how to handle it:

- <u>Carry extras</u> — A pad, a change of underwear, and some wipes in your bag = **lifesavers**!

- <u>Dark-colored clothing</u> — On heavy days, dark leggings or jeans can hide leaks.

- <u>Wrap a sweater around your waist</u> — A classic move when you're in a pinch!

Period Hygiene & Self-Care

- **Wash daily** — Warm water + mild soap = fresh and clean! 🧼

- **Dispose properly** — Wrap used pads/tampons in toilet paper and throw them in the trash. 🗑️ **Never flush!** 🚽❌ 🗑️

- **Stay comfy** — Cozy clothes, heating pads, and your favorite snack? COZY -AND- COMFY **Yes**, please! 🛋️🍫🍿

Menstrual hygiene is a necessity

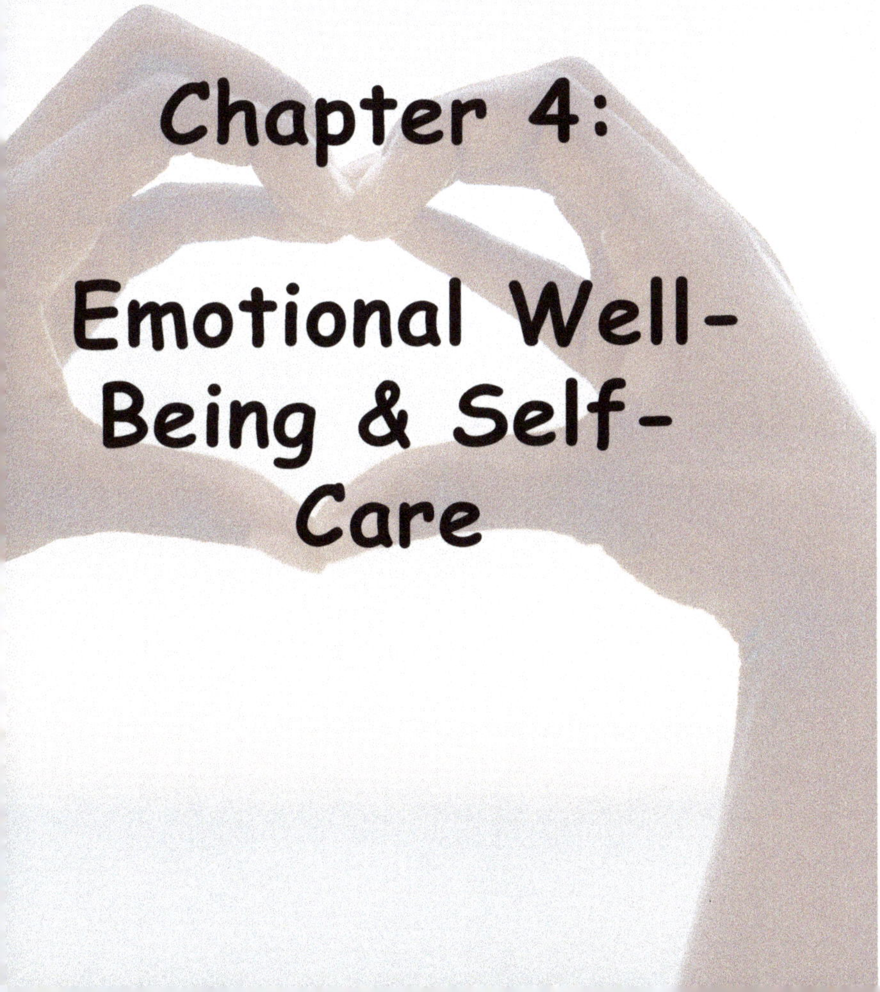

Chapter 4:

Emotional Well-Being & Self-Care

Mood Swings & Emotions

One minute you're laughing at a meme, and the next you're crying over a puppy video—WHAT?!

Welcome to hormone town!

Mood swings are normal, but here's how to handle them:

- **Pause & Breathe** — If you feel overwhelmed, take a deep breath. Count to four, inhale... exhale. 😌
- **Move Your Body** — A short walk or stretch can do wonders!
- **Talk It Out** — Vent to a trusted friend, family member, or even write it down.

Positive Affirmations & Body Positivity

Your body is doing something amazing.

Let's show it some love!

Repeat after me:

- **"I am strong and beautiful just as I am."**

- **"My body is powerful and works exactly as it should."**

- **"I am growing, glowing, and unstoppable!"**

Mindfulness Exercises
for
Cramps & Stress

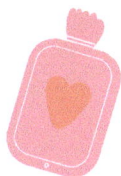

Heat therapy — Use a heating pad or warm towel on your belly.

Gentle yoga — Try child's pose or lying on your back with knees bent.

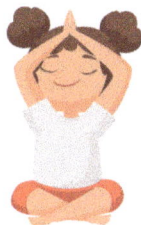

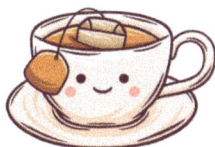

Drink warm tea — Chamomile or ginger tea can ease cramps.

Chapter 5:

HEALTHY HABITS

Foods That Help During Your Period

🥦 **Leafy greens** — Boost iron levels
🍌 **Bananas** — Help with bloating
🍫 Dark chocolate — A tasty mood booster
(yes, really!)

Staying Active & Hydrated
Even if you feel like a couch potato, moving a little can actually make you feel better. And don't forget water—it helps reduce bloating and headaches!

The Importance of Sleep
Your body is working hard, so give it at least 8-10 hours of sleep. Trust me, you'll feel WAY better!

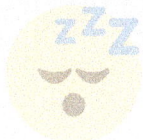

Chapter 6: Talking About It

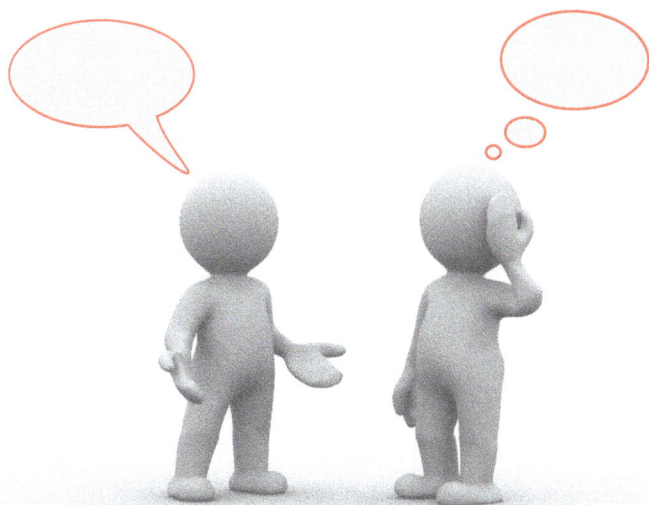

How to Talk to Parents, Caregivers, or Friends

Periods shouldn't be a secret code!
You can simply say:

- "Hey, I think I got my period. Can you help me get some supplies?"
- "I have cramps today, do you have any tips?"

Breaking Myths & Normalizing Period Talk

🚫 Myth: You can't swim on your period.
(False! Tampons and period swimwear exist!)

🚫 Myth: Periods are dirty.
(Nope! They're a natural, healthy process.)

Encouraging Confidence & Self-Advocacy

It's **YOUR** body, and you deserve to feel confident about it. Never be afraid to ask questions or stand up for yourself. Periods are powerful, not shameful!

Chapter 7:
Fun & Interactive Sections

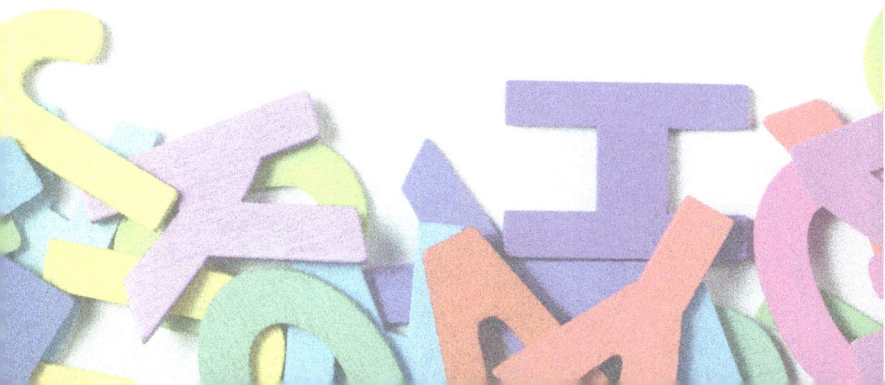

Pages for Tracking Cycles & Moods

Use these pages to jot down when your period starts, how you're feeling, and any cravings or symptoms.

Period Tracker

Tracker ☒

	Jan	Feb	Mar	Apr	May	Jun	Jul	Aug	Sep	Oct	Nov	Dec

Flow ☒

💧 Light

💧💧💧 Medium

💧💧💧💧💧 Heavy

💧 Ovulation

Notes ☒

Cycle Length ☒

Jan	Feb	Mar
Apr	May	Jun
Jul	Aug	Sep
Oct	Nov	Dec

PERIOD TRACKER

J F M A M J J A S

1.
2.
3.
4.
5.
6.
7.
8.
9.
10.
11.
12.
13.
14.
15.
16.
17.
18.
19.
20.
21.
22.
23.
24.
25.
26.
27.
28.
29.
30.
31.

FLOW

Light

Medium

Heavy

NOTE

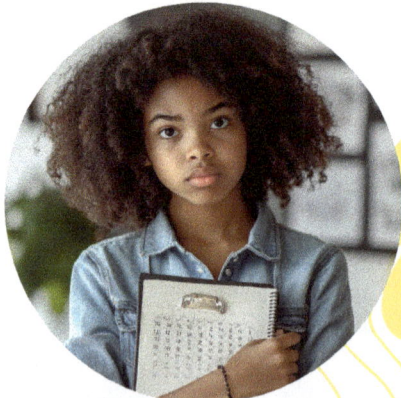

MOOD TRACKER

Flow & Glow

Date:

MY ACTIVITIES

Practice yoga

Take a power nap

Write a journal

Listen to music

Play some games

MY MOOD

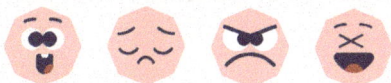

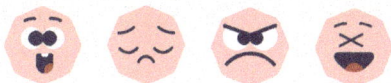

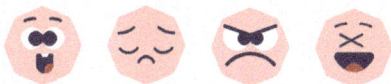

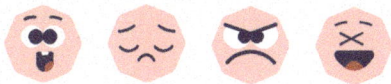

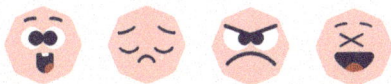

LIST OF MOODS

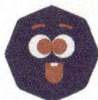
Happy

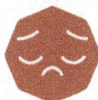
Sad

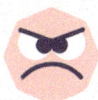
Annoyed

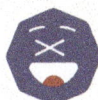
Excited

Date:

MY ACTIVITIES

Practice yoga

Take a power nap

Write a journal

Listen to music

Play some games

MY MOOD

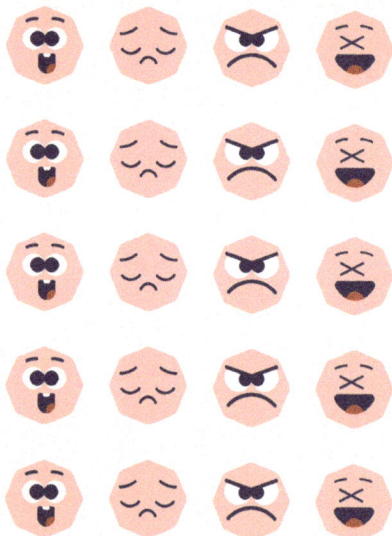

LIST OF MOODS

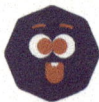
Happy

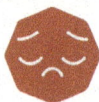
Sad

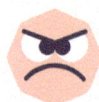
Annoyed

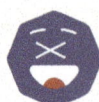
Excited

MY GLOW JOURNAL

NAME : _____

PLAN FOR THE DAY

PRIORITIES

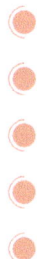

-
-
-
-
-

TODAY'S MOOD:

MEAL TRACKER

BREAKFAST	LUNCH	DINNER

NOTES

AFFIRMATIONS

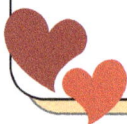

REMINDER

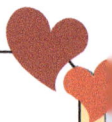

Final Thoughts

Growing up comes with lots of changes, and your period is just one of them.
But guess what?
You are strong, capable, and totally ready for this! 🎉
Now go out there and keep shining, because
you've got this! 💖✨

References

Centers for Disease Control and Prevention. (n.d.). Healthy habits: Menstrual hygiene. Centers for Disease Control and Prevention. https://www.cdc.gov/hygiene/about/menstrual-hygiene.html

Healthline. (2019). 16 Foods to Eat (and Some to Avoid) During Your Period.

KidsHealth. (2021). All About Periods. Nemours Children's Health.

KidsHealth. (2022). Dealing with PMS. Nemours Children's Health.

Nationwide Children's Hospital. Healthy Sleep Habits for Older Children and Teens. https://www.nationwidechildrens.org/family-resources-education/health-wellness-and-safety-resources/helping-hands/healthy-sleep-habits-for-older-children-and-teens

Office on Women's Health, U.S. Department of Health and Human Services. (2021). Your menstrual cycle.https://www.womenshealth.gov/menstrual-cycle

Talking about periods at home. Back to UNICEF.org. (n.d.). https://www.unicef.org/parenting/health/talking-about-periods-at-home

The Flow & Glow Kit
(Practical & Comfort Essentials)

Period Essentials

- Variety of pads (light, regular, heavy)
- A pair of period underwear or pantyliners
- Discreet carrying pouch for school

1. Variety of Pads (Light, Regular, Heavy) 🩸

- Period flow can change from light to heavy, especially in the beginning.
- Having different absorbencies helps prevent leaks and stay comfortable throughout the day.
- Light pads = great for spotting or the last days.
- Regular pads = perfect for most flow days.
- Heavy pads = best for overnight or heavy flow days.

2. A Pair of Period Underwear or Pantyliners 🩲

- Period underwear is reusable, comfy, and absorbs leaks without needing an extra pad.
- Pantyliners are great for light flow days or backup protection with tampons or period cups.

Both help with confidence and freshness throughout the day!

3. Discreet Carrying Pouch for School 👝

- A small pouch makes carrying period products private and stress-free.
- Helps keep supplies organized and easy to grab when needed.
- Can also hold wipes, an extra pair of underwear, and pain relief items.

Self-Care Items

- Small heating pad or reusable heat pack
- Herbal tea or hot chocolate mix for comfort

These self-care items in the menstrual kit help provide comfort, relaxation, and relief during a preteen's period:

- **Small heating pad or reusable heat pack** – Helps soothe cramps and muscle tension by relaxing the abdominal muscles and improving blood flow. A must-have for period comfort! 🩹🧖‍♀️
- **Herbal tea or hot chocolate mix** – Warm drinks like chamomile, peppermint, or ginger tea can ease bloating, cramps, and stress. Hot chocolate is a cozy, mood-boosting treat! ☕🍫

Emergency Supplies

- Stain remover wipes or pen
- Small pack of tissues

The items listed under "Emergency Supplies" in a preteen menstrual kit are meant to help manage unexpected situations and maintain comfort and hygiene:

1. **Stain remover wipes or pen:**
These are for quickly cleaning up any menstrual accidents on clothing, helping to prevent stains and avoid embarrassment if something happens unexpectedly.

2. **Small pack of tissues:**
Tissues are handy for cleaning up or freshening up when needed, especially if there are no access to restrooms with soap and water right away. They're also useful for wiping any excess moisture or for personal hygiene.

These items are all about being prepared and feeling at ease in case of any menstrual-related surprises.

Confidence Boosters

- **Affirmation cards** for self-love and confidence
- A cute, uplifting **sticker**
- Glow **bracelet**
- a mini xWhat's poppin "dat Glow" **lip gloss**
- A handwritten note from the therapist

To get the Flow and Glow packages order at the link below:

Essential Pack:

- Variety of pads (light, regular, heavy)
- Summer's Eve Feminine wipe
- A pair of period underwear or pantyliners
- Wet Wipe
- Herbal tea or hot chocolate mix for comfort
- Small pack of tissues
- Affirmation cards for self-love and confidence
- A cute, uplifting sticker
- Glow bracelet
- You got this mini journal
- A handwritten note from the therapist

Glow Pack:

All of the essential pack items **plus**
- Small heating pad or reusable heat pack
- Lavender Hand sanitizer
- Stain remover wipes or pen
- a mini xWhat's poppin "dat Glow" lip gloss

Contact: authenticexpressions@icloud.com
Shop: AuthentikXpressions on Etsy

Flow and Glow

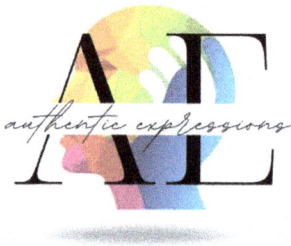

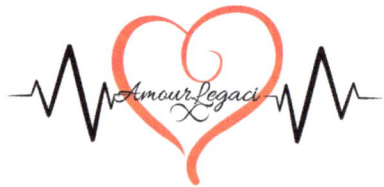

www.ingramcontent.com/pod-product-compliance
Lightning Source LLC
Chambersburg PA
CBHW052025030426
42335CB00026B/3289